The Better Bath vol. 5: Melt and Pour Soaps

I0412075

Written by Lacey Jones

This book contains material protected under International and Federal Copyright Laws and Treaties. Any unauthorized reprint or use of this material is prohibited. No part of this book may be reproduced or transmitted in any form or by any means, electronic or mechanical, including photocopying, recording, or by any information storage and retrieval system without express written permission from the author.

© 2015 All rights reserved.

<u>Disclaimer:</u>

The information contained in this book is for general information purposes only.

While we endeavor to keep the information up to date and correct, we make no representations or warranties of any kind, express or implied, about the completeness, accuracy, reliability, suitability or availability with respect to the book or the information, products, services, or related graphics contained in the book for any purpose. Any reliance you place on such information is therefore strictly at your own risk.

None of the information in this this book is meant to be construed as medical advice. It has not been evaluated by the Food and Drug Administration.

Essential oils are powerful compounds. Consult with a medical professional prior to making changes that could impact your health.

Contents

Introduction

When I first discovered bath bombs, they seemed almost magical to me. I had no clue what caused them to explode into a flurry of fizz and fragrances when tossed into the tub, but I fell in love with them almost instantly. I started buying them from a local boutique, and they weren't cheap, but I was hooked for life. Back then, I was paying $4 to $7 bucks apiece for my bath bombs because they were relatively unheard of and very hard to find, so I had to limit myself to using them once or twice a week.

I'd dabbled in making my own bath products, but I never once considered making bath bombs because the fizzing action seemed so complicated. I thought for sure it would require a precise combination of hard-to-acquire ingredients, so I kept buying them even though they were costing me more than I wanted to pay. Then one day I ran into a nice lady at the boutique, who watched me select several bath bombs and then dropped a bomb of her own on me. I didn't realize it then, but it was one that would change my life.

"You know," she told me. "You're paying a lot of money for those when you can make them at home for a few cents each."

I looked at her in disbelief. There was no way bath bombs were that cheap to make. Besides, they had to be *impossible* to get right. After all, if they were easy to make, everyone would be making them. In retrospect, I should have asked her how to make them then and there, but she'd planted a seed that would change my life. I purchased the bath bombs I'd selected that day, but it was the last day I ever paid full price for bath bombs.

When I got home, I logged into my AOL account and waited for the dial-up to connect (yes, it was that long ago). I typed "bath bomb recipes" into the search engine and was greeted by page after page of results that had nothing to do with bath bombs. Search engines back then weren't what they are now, and the information on obscure items like bath bombs wasn't as readily available as it is today. I was determined to find a recipe for bath bombs, and after an hour or two I finally stumbled upon an Angelfire page that had a single recipe for "fizzing bath balls" on it.

I read the ingredient list and found it hard to believe that this was an actual bath bomb recipe. It only had 5 ingredients and 4 of them were items I already had in the kitchen. The recipe called for the following ingredients:

- **Baking powder.**
- **Citric acid.**
- **Corn Starch.**
- **Water.**
- **Fragrance oil.**

Still doubtful, I put the recipe together (minus the fragrance oil, which I didn't have on hand) and tossed it in the tub. It wasn't perfect like the bath bombs I'd been purchasing, but it fizzed! I did a quick calculation in my head, and it wouldn't cost pennies to make my own bath bombs like the lady at the store had said, but it would be less than a dollar per bath bomb, which was huge savings compared to what I'd been paying.

Little did I know then, but I'd just embarked on a journey that would last the rest of my life. I was hooked on bath bombs and could now afford to use them whenever I wanted to. I was also able to experiment with them and make interesting new fragrances and blends of color that weren't sold in stores.

While bath bombs may seem complicated at first glance, they're actually really easy to make. They'll save you a lot of money when compared to how much it costs to buy them from the store, and you'll have control over what goes into them.

The Main Ingredients: Citric Acid and Baking Soda

There are only two ingredients that are an absolute necessity in bath bombs:

- **Citric acid.**
- **Baking soda.**

That's it. Those two ingredients are the main ingredients, and they're the only ingredients you have to have in order to create a fizzing bath product. When combined dry, citric acid and baking soda don't react to one another, but add water to the mix like you do when you toss a bath bomb into the tub, and you get a semi-violent reaction that creates gas bubbles.

The *baking soda* used in bath bomb recipes is the same run-of-the-mill baking soda used for baking. You've probably got a box or two of it in the pantry, and you might have an open box of it in the fridge to help eliminate bad smells. If you don't have it on-hand, you can buy it at pretty much any grocery store, health food store or drug store in existence. Don't use the open box you have in the fridge…Unless you want your bath to smell like a stinky fridge. You're also going to want to avoid using baking powder instead of baking soda. Baking powder is similar to baking soda, but contains ingredients that aren't necessary in bath bombs and may not be good for your skin.

Citric acid isn't quite as common an ingredient as baking soda, but it can also be purchased at most grocery stores and some health food stores. It's used in some baking recipes, and is used to preserve fruits and other foods. It's a weak organic acid that's commonly found in citrus fruits.

When using baking soda and citric acid in bath bomb recipes, keep the ratio at 2 parts baking soda for every part citric acid used. If you use 1 cup citric acid, you'll need to add 2 cups of baking soda. If you scale up your recipes and are trying to make a big batch, a pound of citric acid will require 2 pounds of baking soda to create an effective bath bomb. It doesn't have to be perfect, but the further away from this ratio you get, the fewer bubbles you're going to have when you toss your bath bombs in the tub.

You might come across some recipes that are improperly labeled as bath bombs, but they don't use citric acid and baking soda. These recipes are usually made up of nut and plant butters and should be labeled as bath melts because they don't have the same fizzing action as the bath bombs do. You'll also see recipes that state cream of tartar is an acceptable replacement for citric acid. In my experience, cream of tartar won't fizz anywhere near as much as baking soda, and you can use it if you have to, but let's be honest here. You're much more likely to have baking soda on-hand, and it's a better choice, so why not stick to the baking soda.

Corn Starch: Make Sure It Floats

Most commercial bath bombs float at the top of the tub, where they spray out a constant stream of bubbles and sometimes send out streams of color. I'm not sure what's used to make the commercial bath bombs float but this same effect can be achieved by adding corn starch to your homemade bath bomb recipe.

Corn starch also adds volume to the bath bombs, bulking them up a bit. It doesn't have much of an effect on the way the bath bombs work unless you add too much. I like to add it in an equal amount to the amount of citric acid that's used in the recipe.

Butters and Oils

Plant and nut butters are another common ingredient found in bath bombs. They make the water in the tub creamier, and adding these butters results in a more luxurious bath time experience. Butters have moisturizing properties that will leave your skin feeling silky smooth when you get out of the tub.

There are a number of butters that can be added to your bath bombs:

- **Avocado butter.** This butter is thick and rich, but it can be a little overbearing when it's the only oil used in the tub.
- **Cocoa butter.** If you're looking for a butter with strong healing and moisturizing properties, cocoa butter is a good choice. It's firm at room temperature and can be added to bath bombs to help firm them up.
- **Illipe butter.** A small amount of Illipe butter can be added to your bath bombs to add moisturizing properties to the bomb. This butter is expensive, but only needs to be used in small quantities to realize its benefits.
- **Shea butter.** This is one of the few butters that doesn't leave an oily sheen behind on your skin. It has moisturizing properties and is a great carrier to help your skin take up essential oils.

This is just a small sampling of the many butters that can be used in bath bombs. You have to be careful not to add to much butter or your bath bomb won't stick together very well and will be prone to melting when temperatures start to climb. There's a fine balance between too little and too much butter, so you've really got to watch how much you're using in your recipes.

You've also got to make sure you balance the amount of butters you use against the amount of carrier oil you add to the recipe. Carrier oils are used to dilute essential oils and make them safe for topical application. When used in bath bomb recipes, carrier oils are there to dilute the essential oils or fragrance oils used in the recipes, and some carrier oils act as dispersing agents that help spread the ingredients in the bath bomb throughout the water column.

The following carrier oils are commonly used in bath bomb recipes:

- **Apricot seed oil.** This oil has a medium viscosity and a slightly-nutty fragrance. It leaves a light oily residue on the skin.
- **Coconut oil.** Virgin coconut oil smells like coconuts and has strong emollient and moisturizing properties. Fractionated coconut oil is a more processed oil that doesn't smell like coconuts, but may contain trace amounts of the chemicals used to fractionate it. Virgin coconut oil feels slightly oily when applied, while fractionated coconut oil doesn't leave much of a residue behind.
- **Grapeseed oil.** Much of the Grapeseed oil sold on the market today is *solvent-extracted*, meaning some sort of chemical solvent is used to remove

the oil from the grape seeds. If you can find pressed Grapeseed oil, it's a better choice. Grapeseed oil smells slightly nutty and leaves behind a light residue.

- **Jojoba oil.** If you've got red, irritated skin, the soothing properties of jojoba oil may be able to provide at least some relief. This "oil" technically isn't an oil at all. It's a wax, but don't let that deter you from using it. It's readily absorbed into the skin and will leave a protective barrier behind.
- **Olive oil.** The thick, viscous nature of virgin olive oil precludes it from being used as the sole oil in a bath bomb recipe, but small amounts of olive oil can be used in skin care recipes. The only type of olive oil you should use is cold-pressed virgin or extra-virgin oil.
- **Sweet almond oil.** This is one of the more popular choices when it comes to carrier oils for bath bomb blends. It has soothing properties and will leave a slightly-oily sheen behind.

When making bath bombs to sell, you have to label them with the types of butters and/or oils you use. People who are allergic to the nuts or fruits the oil came from will also be allergic to the oil. You could be held liable if you fail to label your bath products and they have an allergic reaction.

Another consideration that has to be made is the fact that the oils and butters will leave a residue behind on your skin and on the tub. It can get really slippery, so be careful when getting in and out of the tub.

Fragrance and Essential Oils

While the butters and oils from the previous chapter will add a small amount of fragrance to your bath bombs, using them alone will result in bombs that are, well, a little boring. You're going to want to add something to them to make them smell great.

There are two ways fragrance can be added to bath bombs:

- **Essential oils.**
- **Fragrance oils.**

Essential oils are natural compounds that are derived from plants, and they typically smell like the plants they came from. Eucalyptus oil will smell like eucalyptus trees, rose oil will smell like roses and lavender oil will smell like lavender. It's important to always remember that essential oils are highly-concentrated, and just because they come from plants, that doesn't mean you can use them however you'd like. They're powerful compounds that carry with them a number of properties, some of which are beneficial and some that may not be if they're used improperly.

When used properly, there are a number of essential oils that are beneficial to the vast majority of people who use them, but it's a good idea to consult with your physician prior to adding essential oils to your bath time routine because there are certain oils that shouldn't be combined with certain medications. Also be aware that some oils can exacerbate certain health conditions and there's the risk of an allergic reaction that can range from mild to severe.

Most people are able to use essential oils with no problem as long as they're used in small amounts. They carry a number of therapeutic benefits with them, ranging from being antibacterial and antimicrobial to being able to help you wind down after a long day. It's important you research the oils you plan on using because different oils carry different properties.

While I personally prefer essential oils because they're all-natural, there are certain fragrances that simply can't be achieved through use of essential oils. If you want your bath bombs to smell like clean linen, a tropical paradise or pretty much any fruit other than citrus fruits and maybe apples, you're going to have to use fragrance oils instead of essential oils. *Fragrance oils* are synthetic oils that are designed in a laboratory setting. They don't carry the same therapeutic benefits that essential oils have, but if you're looking to achieve a certain smell that there isn't an essential oil or oil blend available for, they may be your only option.

Other Ingredients

When it comes to other ingredients you can add to bath bombs, the sky's the limit. If it can be broken up into small pieces and it's safe to bathe with, there's probably someone who's added it to a bath bomb.

Here are some of the many ingredients that can be added to bath bombs to spice them up a bit:

- **Bentonite clay.** Composed of volcanic ash, bentonite clay is said to absorb toxins and impurities. It has to be used sparingly in bath bombs because it's really dry and will cause them to crack and split open if you use too much.
- **Dried flowers.** Flowers that have been dried and crumbled are added to bath bombs for aesthetic value. They can be mixed into the "dough" or you can place them in the mold, so that they're stuck to the outside of the bath bomb once it's removed from the mold.
- **Epsom salts.** This is a common ingredient in a number of bath bomb recipes. It helps soften the water in the tub and it helps detoxify the skin and the body.
- **Oatmeal.** Grind oatmeal up and it melts into the tub water, making it feel soft and silky. If you haven't bathed in a bath with ground oatmeal in it, you haven't lived!
- **Powdered milk.** If you've never taken a milk bath, you're missing out. Milk baths are creamy

and luxurious and the lactic acid in the milk helps break down dead skin cells and gently exfoliates the skin.

- **Sea salt.** Sea salts can be used to soften the tub water and they help remedy a number of skin conditions. Sea salts may even provide relief from muscle and joint aches and pains.

You'll also see some recipes that call for *Sodium Lauryl Sulfate (SLS)*. This chemical compound is added strictly to produce more foaming action and probably isn't a great ingredient to add to your homemade bath bombs. If you want to keep them natural, don't use SLS. At the very least, make sure you do a little research before adding it to your bath products. None of the recipes in this book call for it.

Molds: Shaping Your Bath Bombs

You're going to need some sort of mold for your bath bombs. You could take the easy way out and search online for bath bomb molds, but do that and you're really going to limit the shapes and sizes of bath bombs you can make. There's a decent amount of bath bomb molds available today, but there's no reason to limit yourself to just molds that are created specifically for bath bombs.

You can use all sorts of other items as molds, and with a little imagination, the sky's the limit.

Here are some ideas to get you started:

- **A melon baller.**
- **An ice cream scoop.**
- **Candy molds.**
- **Christmas ornaments that can be separated in half.**
- **Cupcake tins.**
- **Easter eggs.**
- **Ice cube trays.**
- **Plastic molds.**
- **Silicon molds.**
- **Stainless steel molds.**

I'm constantly on the lookout for new items I can use as molds. The other day my daughter brought home a few cheap toys from a birthday party. One of the toys was a hollow egg-shaped toy that had interesting shapes on the outside. I talked her into letting me cut it in half and the shapes were on the inside as well. I had to promise her a new toy, but I've now got an awesome mold that makes cool egg-shaped bath bombs!

Coloring Your Bath Bombs

There are a number of colorants that can be used to add color to bath bombs. You can use liquid dyes or powdered colors, but you've got to make sure they're safe for contact with your skin and won't discolor your skin or your tub. Whatever colorant you choose, make sure you only use a small amount and don't overdo it. A little bit of dye goes a long way!

Some companies sell special colorants that are intended for use with bath bombs. These dyes are highly-concentrated and it usually only takes a couple drops to achieve the color you're looking for. They're usually formulated so they won't set off the fizzing reaction between the baking soda and the citric acid when you add them to the bath bomb mix.

You've probably seen bath bombs that are marbled with different colors or layered with colors stacked one on top of the other. This effect is fairly easy to achieve. You'll have to separate your mix into several piles, one for each color. When you're packing it into the mold, pack a small amount of each color at a time. You can pack it in even layers or you can do it unevenly to achieve a marbled look.

Another cool trick is to fill a mold halfway up with mix and then create a well in the middle with your thumb. Fill the well you created with a different color. This color won't show up in the tub until the bath bomb has almost exhausted itself.

Gather Your Supplies

In addition to the rest of the items we've discussed, you're going to need some additional supplies. Here are the items you're going to want to have on-hand before you get started making bath bombs:

- **A rubber spatula.**
- **A spray bottle full of water or witch hazel.** You're going to mist water or witch hazel onto the bath bomb mix until it's damp enough to be moldable.
- **Eye protection.**
- **Glass bowls.**
- **Gloves.**

Make sure you wear gloves and eye protection the entire time you're making bath bombs. Most of the materials you're going to be working with won't cause permanent damage if they get in your eye, but they can definitely irritate your eyes and cause temporary issues. As far as the gloves go, you're going to be mixing the bath bomb mix with your hands. You don't want your skin to be in constant contact with the essential oils and other stuff you're adding to the mix. Also, citric acid stings when it comes in contact with a break in the skin. Trust me on this one!

The Basic Bath Bomb

Let's start with a basic bath bomb. I don't recommend actually making this bath bomb for use unless you want to practice making a batch before you move on to bigger and better things.

This basic recipe is a great jumping off point for future experimentation! Add essential oils and colorants to it and you'll have a functional bath bomb.

Ingredients:
2 cups baking soda
1 cup citric acid
1 cup cornstarch

1 tablespoon coconut oil
1 tablespoon cocoa butter
A spray bottle with water or witch hazel

Directions:

1. Melt the coconut oil and cocoa butter.
2. Combine the baking soda, citric acid and cornstarch and mix until thoroughly blended.
3. Add the oil and butter mix to the dry ingredients and use your hands to knead it in. It has to be completely incorporated. Break up any lumps that form.
4. Lightly mist the mixture with water or witch hazel and work it in with your hands. Keep lightly misting the mixture and working it in until it feels like damp sand and is moldable.

5. Press the mixture into your bath bomb molds. It needs to be packed in firmly.
6. After a couple minutes, the bath bomb can be removed from the mold and left to dry.

The Sea Salt Fizzy

This fizzy takes the basic bath bomb and adds an outer crust of sea salt to it. It's still somewhat basic when it comes to fragrance, so feel free to add your favorite essential oil or fragrance oil to the mix.

I like to use colored sea salts to add character to the bath bomb. One of my personal favorites is Himalayan Pink Salt, which has a natural pink hue to it. If you can't find the color of sea salt you're looking for, you can use your bath bomb colorants to dye the sea salt.

Ingredients:
2 cups baking soda
1 cup citric acid
1 cup cornstarch

1 tablespoon coconut oil
1 tablespoon cocoa butter
A spray bottle with water or witch hazel

1 cup sea salt

Directions:

1. Melt the coconut oil and cocoa butter.
2. Combine the baking soda, citric acid and cornstarch and mix until thoroughly blended.
3. Add the oil and butter mix to the dry ingredients and use your hands to knead it in. It has to be completely incorporated. Break up any lumps that form.

4. Lightly mist the mixture with water or witch hazel and work it in with your hands. Keep lightly misting the mixture and working it in until it feels like damp sand and is moldable.

5. Sprinkle the sea salt liberally into your bath bomb molds.

6. Press the mixture into your bath bomb molds. It needs to be packed in firmly. The sea salt will stick to the bath bombs when you remove them from the molds.

7. After a couple minutes, the bath bomb can be removed from the mold and left to dry.

Tequila Lime Sea Salt Fizzy

Here's a great recipe for those looking to add a little flavor to their bath bombs. This one's a great gift because it looks and smells like you spent hours working on it.

This recipe calls for a few new ingredients. Lime zest can be made by grating or chopping lime peels up into tiny pieces. Lime butter can be made by mixing lime juice with your favorite butter. Lime essential oil can be purchased from most stores that sell essential oils. The tequila is optional, but I like to use it to give this recipe some authenticity. After all, what good is a tequila lime bath bomb that doesn't have a bit of tequila added?

Ingredients:
2 cups baking soda
1 cup citric acid
1 cup cornstarch
2 tablespoons lime zest

1 tablespoon coconut oil
1 tablespoon cocoa butter
1 tablespoon lime butter
10 to 15 drops lime essential oil

A spray bottle with tequila

1 cup green sea salt

Directions:

1. Melt the coconut oil, cocoa butter and the lime butter and stir them together.
2. Let them cool a bit and stir the lime essential oil in.
3. Combine the lime zest, baking soda, citric acid and cornstarch and mix until thoroughly blended.
4. Add the oil and butter mix to the dry ingredients and use your hands to knead it in. It has to be completely incorporated. Break up any lumps that form.
5. Lightly mist the mixture with tequila and work it in with your hands. Keep lightly misting the mixture and working it in until it feels like damp sand and is moldable.
6. Sprinkle the sea salt liberally into your bath bomb molds.
7. Press the mixture into your bath bomb molds. It needs to be packed in firmly. The sea salt will stick to the bath bombs when you remove them from the molds.
8. After a couple minutes, the bath bomb can be removed from the mold and left to dry.

Lavender Salt Bomb

Lavender essential oil is one of my favorite essential oils to use in bath products because it's one of the safest essential oils around. The fragrance of lavender is soothing, and lavender oil has a number of skin care properties associated with it, making it a good choice for bath products.

This recipe calls for purple sea salt. I used to have a local supplier I was able to buy it from, but they haven't had any in stock lately. Now, I take a small amount of bath product safe dye and stir it into white sea salt to get the lavender effect I'm looking for. I also like to add a few drops of lavender essential oil to the sea salt, so my bath bombs smell great straight out of the package! The dried lavender added to this recipe is there for aesthetic value, but can make the tub a little messy. You can leave it out of the recipe if you'd like.

Ingredients:
2 cups baking soda
1 cup citric acid
1 cup cornstarch

1 tablespoon coconut oil
1 tablespoon cocoa butter
10 to 15 drops lavender essential oil

A spray bottle with water or witch hazel

½ cup purple sea salt
½ cup dried lavender

Directions:

1. Melt the coconut oil and cocoa butter and stir them together.
2. Let them cool a bit and stir the lavender essential oil in.
3. Combine the baking soda, citric acid and cornstarch and mix until thoroughly blended.
4. Add the oil and butter mix to the dry ingredients and use your hands to knead it in. It has to be completely incorporated. Break up any lumps that form.
5. Lightly mist the mixture with water (or witch hazel) and work it in with your hands. Keep lightly misting the mixture and working it in until it feels like damp sand and is moldable.
6. Crumble the dried lavender into small pieces. Combine the sea salt and lavender. Sprinkle the sea salt and lavender liberally into your bath bomb molds.
7. Press the mixture into your bath bomb mold. It needs to be packed in firmly. The sea salt will stick to the bath bombs when you remove them from the molds.
8. After a couple minutes, the bath bomb can be removed from the mold and left to dry.

Epsom Salt Bomb

While Epsom salt technically isn't a sea salt, I'm going to include this recipe in this section because it fits better here than anywhere else. Epsom salt is a good addition to bath bombs because it helps soften the water in the tub and it has detoxifying properties.

Fragrance is left up to you for this recipe. Use your favorite essential oil or fragrance oil.

Ingredients:
2 cups baking soda
1 cup citric acid
½ cup cornstarch
½ cup Epsom salt

1 tablespoon coconut oil
1 tablespoon cocoa butter

A spray bottle with water or witch hazel

Directions:

1. Melt the coconut oil and cocoa butter and stir them together.
2. Combine the baking soda, citric acid, Epsom salt and cornstarch and mix until thoroughly blended.
3. Add the oil and butter mix to the dry ingredients and use your hands to knead it in. It has to be completely incorporated. Break up any lumps that form.
4. Lightly mist the mixture with water (or witch hazel) and work it in with your hands. Keep lightly misting

the mixture and working it in until it feels like damp sand and is moldable.

5. Press the mixture into your bath bomb mold. It needs to be packed in firmly.

6. After a couple minutes, the bath bomb can be removed from the mold and left to dry.

Oatmeal Bath Bombs

Add ground oatmeal to your bathwater and something *magical* happens. As long as you grind it up small enough, the oatmeal will melt into the tub water, creating a smooth, luxurious bath that leaves your skin feeling supple and healthy.

This recipe doesn't smell much on its own, so you'll need to add your favorite essential or fragrance oil to the mix.

Ingredients:
2 cups baking soda
1 cup citric acid
1 cup cornstarch
1 cup ground oats

1 tablespoon coconut oil
1 tablespoon cocoa butter

A spray bottle with water or witch hazel

Directions:

1. Melt the coconut oil and cocoa butter and stir them together.
2. Combine the baking soda, citric acid, cornstarch and ground oats and mix until thoroughly blended.
3. Add the melted butter mix to the dry ingredients and use your hands to knead it in. It has to be completely incorporated. Break up any lumps that form.

4. Lightly mist the mixture with water (or witch hazel) and work it in with your hands. Keep lightly misting the mixture and working it in until it feels like damp sand and is moldable.
5. Press the mixture into your bath bomb mold. It needs to be packed in firmly.
6. After a couple minutes, the bath bomb can be removed from the mold and left to dry.

Honey Oatmeal Bombs

The honey oatmeal bomb recipe takes the previous recipe and builds on it by adding raw honey to the mix. Raw honey is soothing to the skin and has antibacterial properties. Don't worry about it making your skin feel sticky…The raw honey melts right into the bath water and you don't even notice it's in there.

I like to add several drops of natural honey fragrance oil to this recipe to make it smell sweeter.

Ingredients:
2 cups baking soda
1 cup citric acid
1 cup cornstarch
1 cup ground oats

1 tablespoon coconut oil
1 tablespoon Shea butter
2 tablespoons raw honey
1 tablespoon natural honey fragrance

A spray bottle with water or witch hazel

Directions:

1. Melt the coconut oil and Shea butter and stir them together. Let the mixture cool for a little while and stir the raw honey and honey fragrance oil into the butter/oil mix.
2. Combine the baking soda, citric acid, cornstarch and ground oats and mix until thoroughly blended.

3. Add the melted butter mix to the dry ingredients and use your hands to knead it in. It has to be completely incorporated. Break up any lumps that form.
4. Lightly mist the mixture with water (or witch hazel) and work it in with your hands. Keep lightly misting the mixture and working it in until it feels like damp sand and is moldable.
5. Press the mixture into your bath bomb mold. It needs to be packed in firmly.
6. After a couple minutes, the bath bomb can be removed from the mold and left to dry.

Powdered Milk Fizzies

Add powdered milk to your bath water and you'll end up with a bath that gently exfoliates your skin thanks to the lactic acid in the milk. It helps break down the dead skin cells, exposing the fresh skin beneath.

This recipe doesn't have any fragrance added, so feel free to use your favorite essential oil blends. Try adding honey and honey fragrance, oatmeal and powdered oats for a wonderful and relaxing bath that smells great.

Ingredients:
2 cups baking soda
1 cup citric acid
1 cup cornstarch
1 cup powdered milk

1 tablespoon coconut oil
1 tablespoon Shea butter

A spray bottle with water or witch hazel

Directions:

1. Melt the coconut oil and Shea butter and stir them together.
2. Combine the baking soda, citric acid, powdered milk and cornstarch and mix until thoroughly blended.
3. Add the melted butter mix to the dry ingredients and use your hands to knead it in. It has to be completely incorporated. Break up any lumps that form.

4. Lightly mist the mixture with water (or witch hazel) and work it in with your hands. Keep lightly misting the mixture and working it in until it feels like damp sand and is moldable.
5. Press the mixture into your bath bomb mold. It needs to be packed in firmly.
6. After a couple minutes, the bath bomb can be removed from the mold and left to dry.

Mint Fizzies

This bath bomb comes with a warning! Peppermint essential oil is a powerful oil that isn't well-tolerated by all people. Peppermint oil creates a sensation similar to vapor rub when it comes in contact with the skin, and the more you use, the more intense the sensation gets. The first time I used it, I was new to using essential oils and I overdid it with the peppermint oil. Let's just say it made for a very uncomfortable bath.

When used in small amounts, most people are able to enjoy the many therapeutic benefits it carries with it. It's good for the skin and has been used as a home remedy for all sorts of skin problems.

Ingredients:
2 cups baking soda
1 cup citric acid
1 cup cornstarch

1 tablespoon coconut oil
1 tablespoon sweet almond oil
10 to 15 drops of peppermint essential oil
A few drops of bath product safe red colorant

A spray bottle with water or witch hazel

Directions:

1. Melt the coconut oil and stir the sweet almond oil into it until they're combined.

2. Add the colorant and stir it in.
3. Let the mixture cool for a bit and stir the peppermint essential oil into it.
4. Combine the baking soda, citric acid and cornstarch and mix until thoroughly blended.
5. Add the oil mix to the dry ingredients and use your hands to knead it in. It has to be completely incorporated. Break up any lumps that form.
6. Lightly mist the mixture with water (or witch hazel) and work it in with your hands. Keep lightly misting the mixture and working it in until it feels like damp sand and is moldable.
7. Press the mixture into your bath bomb mold. It needs to be packed in firmly.
8. After a couple minutes, the bath bomb can be removed from the mold and left to dry.

Citrus Bombs

Citrus bombs use citrus essential oils for fragrance. There are a number of citrus essential oils that can be used, including lemon, lime, grapefruit and Bergamot. Citrus essential oils are good for the skin, and they have a light, refreshing fragrance that will leave you feeling ready to tackle anything that comes your way.

Be aware that some citrus oils are phototoxic and can cause a reaction when they're applied to the skin and you go out in the sun.

Ingredients:
2 cups baking soda
1 cup citric acid
1 cup cornstarch

1 tablespoon coconut oil
2 tablespoons Shea butter
10 to 15 drops of citrus essential oil

A spray bottle with water or witch hazel

Directions:

1. Melt the coconut oil and Shea butter and stir them together until they're combined.
2. Let the mixture cool for a bit and stir the citrus essential oil into it.
3. Combine the baking soda, citric acid and cornstarch and mix until thoroughly blended.

4. Add the oil/butter mix to the dry ingredients and use your hands to knead it in. It has to be completely incorporated. Break up any lumps that form.

5. Lightly mist the mixture with water (or witch hazel) and work it in with your hands. Keep lightly misting the mixture and working it in until it feels like damp sand and is moldable.

6. Press the mixture into your bath bomb mold. It needs to be packed in firmly.

7. After a couple minutes, the bath bomb can be removed from the mold and left to dry.

Lemon Lime Bombs

I used to call this recipe "7-Up Bombs," but I decided to change the name because of trademark concerns. Toss one of these bombs into the tub and climb in, and it really does feel like you're sitting in a tub full of soda.

Ingredients:
2 cups baking soda
1 cup citric acid
1 cup cornstarch

1 tablespoon coconut oil
2 tablespoons Shea butter
5 to 10 drops lemon essential oil
5 to 10 drops lime essential oil
A few drops of green colorant

A spray bottle with water or witch hazel

Directions:

1. Melt the coconut oil and Shea butter and stir them together until they're combined.
2. Add a few drops the green bath product safe colorant and stir it in.
3. Let the mixture cool for a bit and stir the lemon and lime essential oil into it.
4. Combine the baking soda, citric acid and cornstarch and mix until thoroughly blended.

5. Add the oil/butter mix to the dry ingredients and use your hands to knead it in. It has to be completely incorporated. Break up any lumps that form.

6. Lightly mist the mixture with water (or witch hazel) and work it in with your hands. Keep lightly misting the mixture and working it in until it feels like damp sand and is moldable.

7. Press the mixture into your bath bomb mold. It needs to be packed in firmly.

8. After a couple minutes, the bath bomb can be removed from the mold and left to dry.

Cinnamon Orange Fizzies

This recipe can be made without the cinnamon and you'll have plain old orange fizzies, but I really like the way the cinnamon complements the fragrance of the orange essential oil. I used cinnamon fragrance oil in this recipe instead of cinnamon essential oil because the essential oil is really strong and can irritate the skin.

Ingredients:
2 cups baking soda
1 cup citric acid
1 cup cornstarch

1 tablespoon coconut oil
2 tablespoons Shea butter
10 to 15 drops of orange essential oil
5 drops of cinnamon fragrance oil
A few drops of orange colorant

A spray bottle with water or witch hazel

Directions:

1. Melt the coconut oil and Shea butter and stir them together until they're combined.
2. Let the mixture cool for a bit and stir the orange essential oil and the cinnamon fragrance oil into it.
3. Stir a few drops of orange colorant into the butter/oil blend.
4. Combine the baking soda, citric acid and cornstarch and mix until thoroughly blended.

5. Add the oil/butter mix to the dry ingredients and use your hands to knead it in. It has to be completely incorporated. Break up any lumps that form.

6. Lightly mist the mixture with water (or witch hazel) and work it in with your hands. Keep lightly misting the mixture and working it in until it feels like damp sand and is moldable.

7. Press the mixture into your bath bomb mold. It needs to be packed in firmly.

8. After a couple minutes, the bath bomb can be removed from the mold and left to dry.

Tropical Bath Bombs

These bath bomb recipes call for a variety of ingredients that will leave you feeling like you're bathing in a tropical paradise. We start off with a basic recipe that you can tailor to suit your needs and then move on to a handful of specific recipes you can make that have various tropical themes.

These are some of my favorite recipes…Mai Tais, of course, are optional!

Ingredients:
2 cups baking soda
1 cup citric acid
1 cup cornstarch

1 tablespoon coconut oil
2 tablespoons mango butter
10 to 15 drops of your favorite tropical fragrance oil

A spray bottle with water or witch hazel

Directions:

1. Melt the coconut oil and mango butter and stir them together until they're combined.
2. Let the mixture cool for a bit and stir the fragrance oil into it.
3. Combine the baking soda, citric acid and cornstarch and mix until thoroughly blended.

4. Add the oil/butter mix to the dry ingredients and use your hands to knead it in. It has to be completely incorporated. Break up any lumps that form.
5. Lightly mist the mixture with water (or witch hazel) and work it in with your hands. Keep lightly misting the mixture and working it in until it feels like damp sand and is moldable.
6. Press the mixture into your bath bomb mold. It needs to be packed in firmly.
7. After a couple minutes, the bath bomb can be removed from the mold and left to dry.

Coconut Bombs

To me, there's nothing that screams "tropical" louder than the fragrance of coconut. Close your eyes and breathe deeply and pretend you're sitting on a beach somewhere sipping coconut water out of a coconut.

Try adding pineapple fragrance oil to this recipe to create coconut pineapple bombs!

Ingredients:
2 cups baking soda
1 cup citric acid
1 cup cornstarch

1 tablespoon coconut oil
2 tablespoons mango butter
10 to 15 drops of coconut fragrance oil
½ cup white melt and pour soap
½ cup shredded coconut

A spray bottle with water or witch hazel

Directions:

1. Melt the coconut oil and mango butter and stir them together until they're combined.
2. Let the mixture cool for a bit and stir the coconut fragrance oil into it.
3. Combine the baking soda, citric acid and cornstarch and mix until thoroughly blended.

4. Add the oil/butter mix to the dry ingredients and use your hands to knead it in. It has to be completely incorporated. Break up any lumps that form.

5. Lightly mist the mixture with water (or witch hazel) and work it in with your hands. Keep lightly misting the mixture and working it in until it feels like damp sand and is moldable.

6. Press the mixture into your bath bomb mold. It needs to be packed in firmly.

7. After a couple minutes, the bath bomb can be removed from the mold and left to dry.

8. While the bath bomb is drying, melt the melt and pour soap in the microwave. Melt it for 20 to 30 seconds at a time until it's melted. Be careful…The soap will be really hot and can burn you.

9. Let the soap cool for a few minutes. Dip half of each of the bath bombs into the melted soap and then roll them around in the shredded coconut. The coconut will stick to the soap.

10. Let the bath bombs dry until the soap has completely dried before storing them.

Fruit Punch Bombs

This recipe combines three fruity fragrances to create a bath bomb that smells similar to fruit punch. Feel free to add and remove fruit fragrances as you see fit. There are fragrance oils available for pretty much any fruit you can imagine!

Ingredients:
2 cups baking soda
1 cup citric acid
1 cup cornstarch

1 tablespoon coconut oil
2 tablespoons mango butter
5 drops mango fragrance oil
10 drops apricot fragrance oil
10 drops pineapple fragrance oil
10 drops banana fragrance oil

A spray bottle with water or witch hazel

Directions:

1. Melt the coconut oil and mango butter and stir them together until they're combined.
2. Let the mixture cool for a bit and stir the fragrance oils into it.
3. Combine the baking soda, citric acid and cornstarch and mix until thoroughly blended.

4. Add the oil/butter mix to the dry ingredients and use your hands to knead it in. It has to be completely incorporated. Break up any lumps that form.

5. Lightly mist the mixture with water (or witch hazel) and work it in with your hands. Keep lightly misting the mixture and working it in until it feels like damp sand and is moldable.

6. Press the mixture into your bath bomb mold. It needs to be packed in firmly.

7. After a couple minutes, the bath bomb can be removed from the mold and left to dry.

Chocolate-Dipped Banana Fizzy

Once you've tried this bath bomb, you may never want to use another bath bomb again! This is one of my personal favorite fragrances. I just wish there was a banana essential oil available, so this recipe could be all-natural.

Ingredients:
2 cups baking soda
1 cup citric acid
1 cup cornstarch
¼ cup cocoa powder

1 tablespoon coconut oil
2 tablespoons cocoa butter
10 to 15 drops of banana fragrance oil

A spray bottle with water or witch hazel

Directions:

1. Melt the coconut oil and cocoa butter and stir them together until they're combined.
2. Let the mixture cool for a bit and stir the banana fragrance oil into it.
3. Combine the baking soda, citric acid, cocoa powder and cornstarch and mix until thoroughly blended.
4. Add the oil/butter mix to the dry ingredients and use your hands to knead it in. It has to be completely incorporated. Break up any lumps that form.
5. Lightly mist the mixture with water (or witch hazel) and work it in with your hands. Keep lightly misting

the mixture and working it in until it feels like damp sand and is moldable.

6. Press the mixture into your bath bomb mold. It needs to be packed in firmly.

7. After a couple minutes, the bath bomb can be removed from the mold and left to dry.

Glitter Bombs

OK, I've got to admit that getting out of the tub covered in glitter isn't really my favorite thing to do, but everyone I've made these bath bombs for has absolutely loved them. Keep in mind that the smaller the pieces of glitter you use, the more you're going to have stuck to you when you get out of the bath.

The fragrance used for this recipe is up to you.

Ingredients:
2 cups baking soda
1 cup citric acid
1 cup cornstarch
3 tablespoons glitter

1 tablespoon coconut oil
2 tablespoons Shea butter
10 to 15 drops of your favorite essential or fragrance oil

A spray bottle with water or witch hazel

Directions:

1. Melt the coconut oil and Shea butter and stir them together until they're combined.
2. Let the mixture cool for a bit and stir the essential or fragrance oil into it.
3. Combine the baking soda, citric acid and cornstarch and mix until thoroughly blended. Stir the glitter into the mix.

4. Add the oil/butter mix to the dry ingredients and use your hands to knead it in. It has to be completely incorporated. Break up any lumps that form.

5. Lightly mist the mixture with water (or witch hazel) and work it in with your hands. Keep lightly misting the mixture and working it in until it feels like damp sand and is moldable.

6. Press the mixture into your bath bomb mold. It needs to be packed in firmly.

7. After a couple minutes, the bath bomb can be removed from the mold and left to dry.

Bonus Recipe: Toilet Bombs

You don't have to limit your use of bath bombs to the bath. You can also make cleansing toilet bombs that fizz and bubble while cleaning and disinfecting the toilet. While they don't exactly make cleaning the toilet fun, they do make it marginally more interesting, and the essential oils used in this recipe smell great.

Note that I used a lot more essential oil in this recipe than I do in the bath bomb recipes. That's because this recipe doesn't come in contact with your skin, and I wanted to up the disinfecting powers of the toilet bombs. Don't mix these up with your bath bombs and accidentally throw one in the tub!

Ingredients:
2 cups baking soda
1 cup citric acid
1 cup cornstarch

15 drops of lavender essential oil
20 drops of peppermint essential oil
15 drops of lemon essential oil

A spray bottle with water or witch hazel

Directions:

1. Combine the baking soda, citric acid and cornstarch and mix until thoroughly blended.
2. Stir the essential oils into the mix.

3. Lightly mist the mixture with water (or witch hazel) and work it in with your hands. Keep lightly misting the mixture and working it in until it feels like damp sand and is moldable.
4. Press the mixture into your bath bomb mold. It needs to be packed in firmly.
5. After a couple minutes, the toilet bomb can be removed from the mold and left to dry.

www.ingramcontent.com/pod-product-compliance
Lightning Source LLC
Chambersburg PA
CBHW070625290526
45790CB00002B/993